HOW TO MANAGE GERD

—

GASTROESOPHAGEAL REFLUX DISEASE CAN BE BEATEN

Jacob Rosenberg, MD

ISBN: 150245758X
ISBN-13: 978-1502457585

CONTENT

JACOB ROSENBERG

PREFACE

Gastroesophageal reflux disease (GERD) is very common, and almost all people have at some point had heartburn as a mild symptom of GERD. The symptoms range from the occasional heartburn, e.g. after a high volume dinner, to invalidating symptoms where daily quality of life is severely impaired. In the most extreme cases recurrent lung symptoms, change of voice and even erosion of teeth can be seen. Abdominal pain and chest pain are common complaints that often lead to various diagnostic tests before the right diagnosis can be settled. There are numerous products on the market claiming to alleviate symptoms of GERD, but often with little information on how to use them effectively, and how to position the single product in the jungle of competing products and regimens. The present book will cover the pathophysiology, diagnosis, non-medical as well as medical and surgical treatment options for GERD. There is a therapeutic option for all patients, and control of symptoms of GERD can almost always be accomplished.

Jacob Rosenberg, MD

INTRODUCTION

Gastroesophageal reflux is the name covering the symptoms that can appear when gastric content is flushed upwards into the esophagus and damage or otherwise influence the cell lining in the esophagus. Gastroesophageal reflux disease, also called GERD, and its sequelae is a very common phenomenon in the Western World. Thus, at least 20% of the population has weekly symptoms of reflux and the incidence is increasing. It is important to acknowledge, that this disease can present with very different degrees of severity from the lightest clinical picture without need for medical treatment to very severe and difficult treatable symptoms that cause severe work-related and social problems for the patient. All together gastroesophageal reflux disease may cause significant problems and deterioration of quality of life in many patients.

THE MECHANISM OF REFLUX

The lower esophageal sphincter is the central part of the reflux barrier. The sphincter consists of a 3-4 cm part of the lower esophagus with slightly thickened muscle layers. This area, because of the tonic contraction, is capable of withholding a fully competent reflux barrier, also when the sphincter area is displaced from its normal intraabdominal placement as in a hiatus hernia. There is no tight clinical connection between reflux disease and hiatus hernia, even though many patients with reflux disease do have a hiatus hernia. There are many patients where a hiatus hernia is a random finding and where treatment of neither the hernia nor reflux is not indicated.

The primary cause of reflux is dysfunction of the lower esophageal sphincter because reflux will occur when the pressure in the muscle decreases.

Two types of sphincter dysfunction have been identified. The most important mechanism is an increased occurrence of transient sphincter relaxations that occur especially after meals, probably caused by distention of the stomach. The physiological function behind these relaxations is probably to allow for burping, thus enabling air to escape from the stomach through the esophagus and mouth. The other and much more rare sphincter dysfunction is a continuous low basal pressure in the lower esophageal sphincter. This reflux mechanism is especially seen in patients with esophagitis.

The function of the sphincter can be compromised even more when there is a hiatus hernia where the external support from the crurae of the diaphragm is missing and the sphincter is shortened and positioned in the thoracic pressure environment instead of intraabdominally.

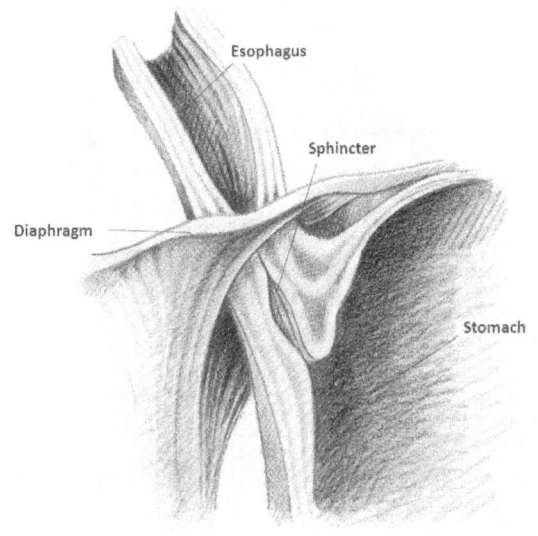

A number of other factors can initiate the reflux: delayed gastric emptying will increase the gastric content and thereby increase the possibility for reflux; decreased salivary secretion and dysmotility in the esophagus will decrease the neutralization of acid reflux material and cause a slow "cleaning" of the esophagus after reflux incidence; decreased resistance of the cell lining in the esophagus against gastric content can give symptoms even at mild incidences of reflux.

Reflux mechanism

The primary cause of reflux is dysfunction of the lower esophageal sphincter.

There is no clear connection between reflux disease and hiatal hernia.

REFLUX DISEASE AND BILE REFLUX

Duodenal content is often present in the esophagus in patients with gastroesophageal reflux disease. There seems to be a connection between the severity of duodeno-gastroesophageal reflux and the severity of the mucosal lesions in the esophagus with the most severe reflux when Barrett's esophagus (see later in this book) is present. Human investigations have, however, shown that bile reflux alone (in patients after gastrectomy) can cause symptoms but no mucosal changes. In patients with reflux disease, acid therefore seems to be the central damaging factor causing mucosal lesions (esophagitis and Barrett's esophagus).

Treatment with proton pump inhibitors will decrease both the degree of acid reflux as well as bile reflux. The mechanism is probably a combination of decrease in the volume of gastric content available for reflux and also the production of a local environment with a pH-value high enough to inactivate the conjugated bile acids that are primarily responsible for the mucosal changes in the esophagus if bile reflux is present.

REFLUX DISEASE AND HELICOBACTER PYLORI

The relationship between reflux disease and helicobacter pylori infection has not been clearly defined. In spite of huge amounts of research data it has not been possible to establish for certain if the infection will protect against reflux, worsen the reflux symptoms and sequelae, or if the two diseases are not connected.

Reflux disease is defined by a defect reflux barrier while smaller changes in the acid secretion probably only have minor importance. The finding of increased acid production after eradication of helicobacter pylori and the epidemiological data showing an increased prevalence of reflux disease and in parallel with this a decreasing prevalence of helicobacter pylori infection have nevertheless given the assumption that helicobacter pylori infection may protect against reflux. However, the evidence for this is not entirely clear.

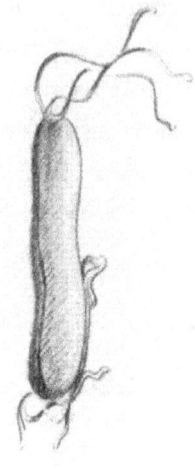

In spite of these problems there seems to be agreement among physicians that patients with helicobacter pylori infection and simultaneous reflux disease that requires continuous treatment with proton pump inhibitors, have a risk of accelerated development of mucosal atrophy in the stomach and that they therefore should receive eradication treatment.

Reflux disease and helicobacter pylori

Patients with helicobacter pylori infection and simultaneous reflux disease necessitating continuous proton pump inhibitor treatment should receive eradication treatment against helicobacter pylori infection.

DIAGNOSIS OF REFLUX DISEASE

The term "gastroesophageal reflux disease" should be used to include all individuals who are exposed to the risk of physical complications from gastroesophageal reflux or who experience clinically significant impairment of health related well-being (quality of life) due to reflux related symptoms, after adequate reassurance of the benign nature of their symptoms.

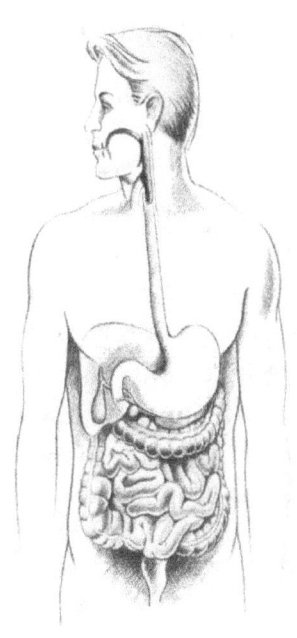

Diagnosis of reflux disease

Anamnesis: Detailed symptom analysis is a central part of the diagnostic process of reflux disease.

Test treatment: The symptom analysis can be expanded and the diagnosis secured by a proton pump inhibitor test treatment for 14 days with evaluation of symptoms before, during and after treatment.

Endoscopy: The majority of patients with reflux disease have no esophagitis at endoscopy.

pH-evaluation: 24 hours pH-evaluation is used primarily in the evaluation of patients, where anti-reflux surgery is considered as a treatment option, but also diagnostically in patients with normal endoscopy and a symptom analysis that is not exclusive for reflux disease or with other atypical symptoms.

SYMPTOM ANALYSIS

A meticulous evaluation of the patient's symptoms is the most important diagnostic tool in the management of patients with reflux disease.

The dominating symptoms are heartburn and regurgitation and it is typical that these symptoms especially present themselves after meals. However, a big group of patients with reflux have reflux when lying down or when bending over, or reflux at physical strain. The term "heartburn" does not describe the symptom complex very good and normally it is necessary to discuss the symptoms in more detail with the patient. Thus, heartburn has nothing to do with the patient's heart, but is more likely described as a burning sensation starting in the upper part of the abdomen or below the lower part of the sternum moving upwards towards the neck and pharynx area.

Careful assessment of patient history that is the most important tool in the diagnosis of reflux disease can be misled by misinterpretation of the word heartburn by the patients. The description of heartburn as "a burning feeling rising from the stomach or lower chest up towards the neck", has been found to make sense to most patients instead of using the word heartburn.

Reflux disease can also give atypical symptoms

such as painful swallowing, harshness, chronic cough, asthma-like symptoms, damage to the teeth, or even angina-like chest-pain.

At the critical symptom analysis it is possible sometimes to reveal other alarm symptoms such as dysphagia, weight loss or bleeding and this will normally indicate subacute gastroscopy.

The patient's quality of life is decreased proportionally to the frequency and severity of heartburn, no matter if esophagitis is present or not. The diagnosis is based on the recurrence of heartburn two or more days per week, since reflux disease is likely to be present if heartburn is a major or sole symptom. Thus, when heartburn is a major or sole symptom gastroesophageal reflux is the cause in at least 75% of individuals. On the other hand, heartburn is the most common symptom of reflux disease occurring in at least 75% of patients, and heartburn that occurs in the absence of definite reflux esophagitis is still most likely due to gastroesophageal reflux.

PROTON PUMP INHIBITOR TEST

In order to increase the diagnostic accuracy of the symptom analysis when typical symptoms are present, it is a good idea to perform a proton pump inhibitor test. At this test a proton pump inhibitor is prescribed in high dosage for a short period of time under close evaluation of symptoms before, during and after this test treatment. A drug for this test treatment could e.g. be esomeprazol 40 mg daily for 2 weeks or even 40 mg twice daily for 2 weeks. Other drugs can also be used, but it is necessary to give the proton pump inhibitor in a high dose for this test period. This diagnostic test is cheap, safe and non-invasive and has a high diagnostic accuracy for reflux disease. If positive response, then the strategy for initial treatment can be followed, as long as no alarm symptoms are present. If alarm symptoms are present, then a proton pump inhibitor test should not be used, and the patient should of course go directly to gastroscopy.

GASTROSCOPY

About 60% of patients with reflux disease have a normal gastroscopy without any signs of esophagitis, and gastroscopy therefore has a limited role as a diagnostic tool in reflux disease. If esophagitis is found at gastroscopy, then it is of course diagnostic for reflux disease, but the absence of esophagitis does not rule out reflux disease. It is important to establish, that the absence of esophagitis does not tell anything at all about the severity of the patient's symptoms, since the whole spectrum from very light to the worst symptoms can be present regardless of the presence of esophagitis at gastroscopy.

Nevertheless, gastroscopy plays an important role in the management of patients with reflux disease because endoscopy is the most sensitive evaluation to diagnose manifestations and complications to reflux disease. If a peptic stricture is found at gastroscopy, it is simple to treat this by balloon dilatation during the same procedure. Control gastroscopy is only rarely indicated unless very severe esophagitis is found at the primary gastroscopy, which hinders the evaluation of the mucosal integrity. Thus, if it has been impossible to see if esophageal malignancy is present, then it is of course indicated to repeat the gastroscopy procedure after effective medical treatment. Usually, the effectiveness of medical treatment is easy to follow by simply following the patient's symptoms. Thus, there is a correlation between the decrease of symptoms and the healing of esophagitis in these patients. Therefore, in a patient with esophagitis it is reasonable to believe, that the esophagitis changes have healed if the patient's symptoms have disappeared.

Indication for gastroscopy:

- **Alarm symptoms:**
  Dysphagia
  Bleeding
  Weight loss
  Anemia
- **Diagnostic problems, e.g. at atypical symptoms (angina-like chest pain, asthma-like symptoms, chronic cough, harshness) after other relevant investigations have been completed.**
- **Preoperatively before antireflux surgery.**
- **Severe chronic reflux: as screening for complications such as strictures, esophagitis and Barrett's esophagus.**

24-HOURS PH-EVALUATION

For this evaluation a pH-electrode is placed in the esophagus with the point of measurement localized 5 cm above the oral border of the lower esophageal sphincter. Localization of the lower esophageal sphincter has been found by esophagus manometry before the pH measurement. At the measurement the total time during the 24-hours evaluation where pH in the esophagus is lower than 4 is registered. The number and duration of reflux episodes are also registered as well as the number of reflux episodes with a duration of more than 5 minutes each. The patient can during the evaluation make notes of the exact timing for symptoms and by this the timely correlation between symptoms and reflux episodes can be mapped as well.

NON-OPERATIVE TREATMENT

Changes in life style

Patients with reflux disease are often recommended to change their life style, but there is only vague evidence for this intervention and no evidence for the life style changes as the single initial treatment against reflux symptos. Patients are typically led to believe, that they can cure themselves by correction of inappropriate life style, but this is a typical misunderstanding. If the negative effects on quality of life by the induced life style changes are taken into account, then it is important to give such recommendations only in areas, where some kind of (low level) evidence is present, and where a change would seem reasonable when taken the patient's previous life style into account.

The typical life style modifications that are recommended are:

Elevated head of the patient's bed
No alcohol
No tobacco
No coffee
Weight loss

Elevated head of the bed:
There has been no effect shown in the typical patient with reflux disease having reflux episodes after meals. However, there may be a subgroup that can clearly describe position related reflux, and in this group it may be a good idea to recommend elevation of the head of the bed.

Tobacco:
Smoking will give an increased number of reflux episodes and a slower eradication of the acid from the esophagus after the reflux episode. A direct beneficial effect of smoking cessation on reflux disease has not been proven, but from a theoretical point of view there seems to be a good reason to advise against smoking in patients with reflux disease.

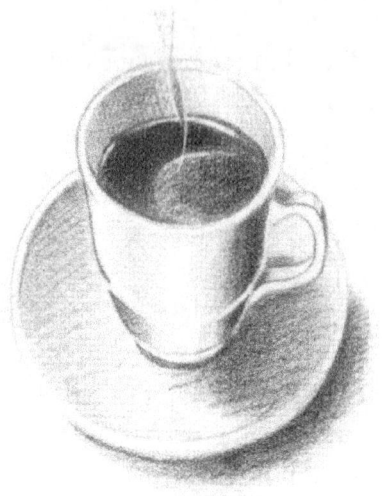

Coffee:
Epidemiologic data have pointed at coffee as an independent risk factor for reflux, but no direct relationship has been proven.

Weight loss:
The ingestion of food with high content of fat will result in an increased number of reflux episodes. However, a study found that a diet with fewer calories giving a weight loss of around 10 kg did not change the patients' symptoms or reflux episodes when evaluated by 24 hours pH-evaluation. Nevertheless, some overweight patients with reflux will achieve symptom control just by losing weight and advice about weight loss in the overweight should therefore, also from a general health point of view, be advised.

General recommendations for life style changes should therefore be much more concessional than previously thought. When that has been said it should be mentioned, that a group of patients can describe a certain life style or ingestion of certain types of food that for certain will worsen their symptoms. It is therefore of course recommended in these patients, that they should avoid these specific worsening factors.

MEDICAL TREATMENT

The principal mechanisms of the most effective medical treatment of reflux disease is a reduction in the gastric acid production causing the intragastric pH to be above 4, especially at times, where reflux symptoms occur. This treatment does not change the tendency for reflux that will still occur, but now with no acid reflux content. However, the natural course of the reflux disease will typically show a high tendency for recurrence if medical treatment is stopped.

It is difficult to compare the different treatment modalities because only few of them have been evaluated in direct comparative studies, and because reflux disease and reflux esophagitis occur in a continuum of all degrees of severity and the different patient samples have not been comparable in the published studies. Nevertheless, there seems to be agreement worldwide about the following principles:

If the different treatment modalities are ranged under the basis of the effect on reflux esophagitis, then antacids are the weakest drugs with a therapeutic gain of only 10% compared with placebo. Antacids can only be given as a stand-alone treatment in the mildest cases, but can also be used as a supplement to other kinds of treatment. The effect of antacids occurs almost immediately after ingestion, but the effect is short-lasting.

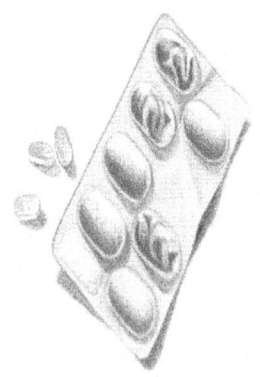

The effect of prokinetics in the treatment of reflux disease has in spite of the apparent good principle been disappointing. The efficiency is at a level comparable to antacids and H_2-receptor antagonists when treating patients with esophagitis.

The effectiveness of H_2-receptor antagonists is only slightly better than the effect of antacids (therapeutic gain 10-24%). The different drugs seem to be comparable and the effectiveness can apparently not be improved by increasing the dose compared with the standard dose.

Only when using proton pump inhibitors it is possible to achieve an almost maximum therapeutic gain (60-75%) compared with placebo. Response to proton pump inhibitor treatment is dose related and there is also a patient group where the intragastric pH cannot be brought over 4 by the use of standard doses. It is important to know the existence of this group of patients because they should be treated with doses sometimes considerably higher than the standard dosing of proton pump inhibitors.

Reflux disease has a very high tendency to reoccur when medical treatment is stopped. It is therefore often necessary to continue medical treatment for a longer period and then at intervals try to reduce the dose. If symptoms reoccur then treatment should be restarted.

Strategy for initial treatment

The initial treatment of patients with reflux disease consists of a thorough explanation of the disease, symptoms and the natural cause of the disease with and without treatment. Changes in life style can be considered, but as mentioned above, the effect is often questionable unless there are specific reasons to change certain types of behavior. Weight loss in overweight patients and smoking sensation in heavy smokers can also from a general point of view be beneficial and will therefore normally be recommended. The group of patients that clearly describes position related reflux can be recommended to elevate the head of the bed when sleeping. The patient is informed about the possibility of self treatment with antacids and H_2-receptor antagonists, which are sold over the counter in most countries. In some countries also proton pump inhibitors are sold over the counter, but it is normally recommended only to use this as over the counter medication after thorough explanation by a specialist.

The purpose of the initial treatment is fast symptom control. The use of the most effective medical treatment is therefore logical and the initial medical treatment should therefore comprise proton pump inhibitor in standard dosing or above.

After 4 weeks treatment it is recommended to stop treatment because a group of patients will not have need for further medical treatment after these initial 4 weeks of treatment with proton pump inhibitors. The patients who obtain prompt symptoms of recurrence after stop of treatment will have a need for long-term treatment with proton pump inhibitors.

Treatment strategy

Aim of initial treatment:

Relief of symptoms as fast as possible and healing of potential underlying esophagitis

Aim of long-term treatment:

To keep the patient free from recurrence with the highest possible quality of life

Strategy for long-term treatment

Most patients with reflux disease will need long-term treatment. It is important to remember, that the natural course of disease in different patients comprises a continuum of all different grades of severity and that long-term treatment therefore should be individualized.

The main principle is to titrate treatment to the lowest effective dose and the cheapest treatment that is still effective for the patient. The target is to keep the patient free from recurrence and with the highest possible quality of life.

If symptoms reoccur after stop of medical treatment after the initial treatment plan with standard dose of proton pump inhibitor, then this treatment should be restarted for another 4 weeks and after this again a titration to the lowest effective dose should be tried. Long-term treatment could comprise standard dose proton pump inhibitor, half dose proton pump inhibitor, proton pump inhibitor on demand, or perhaps a standard dose of H_2-receptor antagonists if this proofs to be effective for the specific patient.

A group of patients will not need constant treatment. These patients are treated with short series with standard doses, and in some cases half standard dose of proton pump inhibitors managed according to symptoms.

JACOB ROSENBERG

Medical treatment

Initial treatment:
Standard dose proton pump inhibitor for 4 weeks and thereafter stop of treatment. If symptoms occur then additional 4 weeks of treatment is initiated, and thereafter the treatment should be titrated to the lowest effective dose and in many patients eventually to no medication

Long-term treatment:
Titration to the cheapest treatment alternative that is still effective against the patient's symptoms

Remember: All different grades of severity of reflux disease can be found and there are therefore numerous different levels of treatment. Thus, some patients can control symptoms with just intermittent treatment and others will not respond to standard dose proton pump inhibitors, and the dose must therefore be increased to a proper clinical effect. Response to proton pump inhibitor treatment is dose dependent

A group of patients with severe reflux disease will not respond to standard dose of proton pump inhibitors. It is very important to know the existence of these patients, and they have to be treated with a gradual increase of the proton pump inhibitor dose to proper clinical effect. This will sometimes imply high doses for the individual patients, and often given twice daily instead of once daily. The typical clinical effect of a single dose of proton pump inhibitor is about 16 hours, and this is why twice daily dosing is indicated if one daily dose is not able to give symptom control 24/7.

Indication for gastroscopy

Alarm symptoms:
Dysphagia
Bleeding
Weight loss
Anemia

Diagnostic problems: e.g. atypical symptoms (angina-like chest pain, asthma-like symptoms, chronic cough, hoarseness) after other relevant investigations have been completed

Preoperatively before anti-reflux surgery: As screening for complications such as strictures, esophagitis and Barrett's esophagus in these patients with severe chronic reflux

COMPLICATIONS TO GASTROESOFAGEAL REFLUX DISEASE

Strategies for Barrett's esophagus

Barrett's esophagus represents a consequence of chronic reflux, where the normal planocellular epithelium in the esophagus is replaced by a specialized cylindrical epithelium with goblet cells, so called intestinal metaplasia. In patients with chronic reflux the prevalence of Barrett's esophagus is about 10% but the incidence is increasing with increasing duration of the reflux disease. Thus, more than 20% of patients with a duration of reflux disease of more than 10 years will have Barrett's esophagus if evaluated by endoscopy.

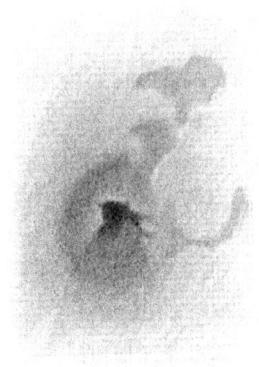

Finding of patients at risk is difficult because an unknown, but probably large group of patients will have Barrett's esophagus actually without any symptoms of gastroesophageal reflux. The importance of this intestinal metaplasia is that the majority of cases of adenocarcinoma (cancer) in the esophagus will develop in areas with intestinal metaplasia. The incidence of adenocarcinoma in the esophagus is increasing rapidly but it is still a relatively rare form of cancer compared with the big cancer diseases such as lung cancer, breast cancer, etc. The risk that a patient with Barrett's esophagus will develop cancer is estimated, based on large prospective series, to be about 30 times higher than in the background population.

The typical Barrett's epithelium is macroscopically visible at endoscopy with a pink area, almost colored like salmon, in the normal esophagus mucosa that is paler, but the final diagnosis is histological after multiple biopsies are taken.

Adenocarcinoma in areas with Barrett's esophagus probably develops after a sequence of changes, beginning with chronic reflux resulting in intestinal metaplasia, followed by dysplasia and finally the development of cancer.

In order to find patients at risk early in the development of the disease and thereby in order to give a better prognosis, patients with Barrett's esophagus should be enrolled in surveillance programs with routine control endoscopies. However, there is not uniform agreement about this around the world. The frequency of these control endoscopies is changed according to the occurrence of dysplasia and the degree of the dysplasia. At every endoscopy multiple biopsies are taken from areas with visible intestinal metaplasia as well as from other areas in the esophagus. The occurrence of intestinal metaplasia will increase the indication for antireflux surgery because especially the short Barrett's segments can actually disappear after laparoscopic fundoplication against reflux disease. It is, however, still uncertain if the combined risk for malignant disease will be decreased after operation, and there are still not data for long-term survival with and without operation. New treatment principles with endoscopic removal of the metaplastic epithelium by e.g. photodynamic treatment, mucosal resection or argon plasma coagulation, which is followed by healing with normal epithelium, seem promising, but it is too early to give final recommendations because we still need data from high quality studies with long-term follow-up.

Proposal for a surveillance program for patients with Barrett's esophagus

No dysplasia:
Control endoscopy every second to third year

Low grade dysplasia:
Control endoscopy every six months for 1 year followed by yearly controls if the dysplasia does not progress to high grade dysplasia

High grade dysplasia:
Either endoscopy controls every 3 months with multiple biopsies or esophageal resection

Strictures in the distal esophagus

Chronic reflux can lead to strictures (so called peptic strictures) in the distal part of the esophagus. The main clinical symptom is dysphagia that can be followed by weight loss and varying degrees of reflux complaints. As in all patients with dysphagia fast endoscopy is important to rule out malignant causes.

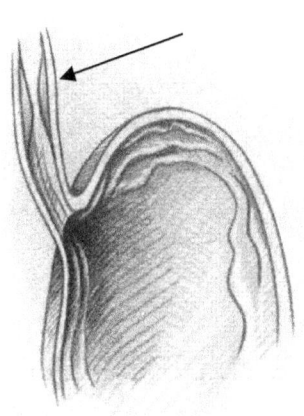

At gastroscopy, biopsies are taken from the stricture and if these are benign, then endoscopic dilatation may be performed at a subsequent endoscopy using a balloon through the gastroscope. It may be necessary to perform with multiple dilatations (multiple gastroscopies) before the dysphagia has disappeared. Continuous proton pump inhibitor treatment is an important part of the treatment regimen to ensure a good final result of treatment with loss of dysphagia. The occurrence of peptic strictures in the distal esophagus is a relative indication for anti-reflux surgery (see below).

Laryngitis

Chronic or recurrent laryngitis, recurrent pneumonias, and asthma-like symptoms can sometimes be an indication for operation if medical treatment is not able to control the symptoms, and if pathological reflux has been verified by pH-measurements. It is, however, not possible for sure to verify if the reflux is the exact cause of the symptoms and thereby the end result of surgery is difficult to predict. It is normally believed in both physicians and surgeons, that the occurrence of laryngitis caused by reflux disease is a rare condition but it is not supported by scientific evidence, which in fact is lacking.

Bleeding

Gastroesophageal reflux disease can sometimes cause bleeding from the esophagus to a degree that the patient presents either with chronic anemia or more rarely with acute bleeding, i.e. haemathemesis and/or melaena. The diagnosis is made at the gastroscopy and the treatment is medical with proton pump inhibitors. The prognosis is good.

OPERATION FOR REFLUX DISEASE

Operative treatment for reflux disease was for years a

rare surgical procedure in the Western World. However, after the introduction of laparoscopic anti-reflux surgery, the situation has changed and the operation can be done by laparoscopy with very low operative morbidity and mortality. Thus, the procedure is in expert surgical centers followed by very low postoperative morbidity, short length of hospital stay (even as day cases), and a very short convalescence period with a high success rate, meaning very good results concerning reflux symptoms after operation. An operation will offer the patient possibility for permanent solution with cessation of reflux of acid from the stomach as well as bile and pancreatic juice. This, combined with the increasing incidence of adenocarcinoma in the distal esophagus and cardia region being strongly associated with chronic reflux, has increased the surgical activity in this area. However, it should of course be emphasized, that the choice of patients for surgery, the operation itself and the adequate postoperative treatment of these patients are specialized tasks only for surgeons with a special interest in this clinical area. Thus, the operative activity around the world is typically centralized to few centers in a certain region.

The operation is performed under general anesthesia as a laparoscopic procedure with 5 laparoscopic "ports" that enter the abdomen through the abdominal wall, each causing wounds at about 1 cm in length. For the trained surgeon conversion to open surgery is extremely rare.

The surgical principles are:

The upper part of the stomach and the lower part of the esophagus are mobilized whereby a possible hiatal hernia is removed (whereby the hernia involving part of the cardia and stomach is placed in the abdomen instead of above the diaphragm). The lower part of the esophagus including the sphincter is also placed intraabdominally.

Suturing by one or more sutures making a cruraplasty diminishes the hiatus. This will make the hiatus fit in size to the esophagus now with normal anatomical placement.

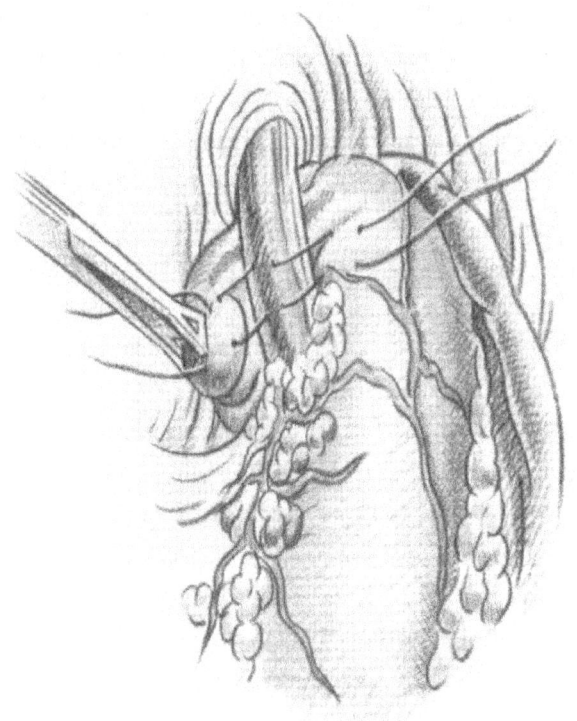

The fundus of the stomach is folded and sutured around the lower part of the esophagus thus making a 1.5 cm wide "manchetta" with typically 2 sutures. In this way the fundus is wrapped around the lower part of the esophagus making a fundoplasty.

The length of hospital stay after the operation is typically one day with a range from 0 to several days depending on local traditions. The average convalescence time after operation is typically about 2 weeks, but with very wide differences primarily based on differences in physical demands in the patient's normal daily life as well as local traditions around the World. There are very few surgical as well as medical complications, but postoperative minor complaints are common. These complaints include transient dysphagia in about a third of the patients. The dysphagia is often short lasting, but can be present for the first 4 to 8 weeks after operation. Shortly after surgery it is possible to see air distension in the stomach after eating (bloating). The cause of this is typically a habit of too fast intake of food and at the same time a lacking possibility to burp. It will disappear when the patient is informed properly about the phenomena and what the cause is. The lack of ability to burp and to throw up is seen during the first month after surgery in about half of the patients. Only the lacking ability to burp may give long term problems because of an increased amount of air in the bowels with resulting increased flatulence. The problems, however, will typically lessen during the first month after surgery.

The classical indication for anti-reflux surgery is an insufficient response to medical treatment. However, nowadays with the very effective modern medical treatment with highly effective proton pump inhibitors, this group is diminished, but there is still a small group of patients with incomplete or unsatisfying effects of medical treatment, even at very high doses. There are also some, especially younger patients, who in spite of quite good symptom control during optimal medical treatment, do not want life-long medical treatment. These patients are in many places also operated with good results. The treatment of complications to chronic reflux such as peptic strictures and Barrett has been improved after treatment with proton pump inhibitors, but the occurrence of peptic strictures and Barrett are still relative indications for antireflux surgery.

Chronic reflux causing respiratory complications such as recurrent pneumonias, asthma-like symptoms, chronic cough and laryngitis is a good indication for surgery. The occurrence of respiratory complications to chronic reflux is probably rare and it is very difficult to choose these patients correctly for surgery, since we don't have any examinations that with certainty can confirm micro-aspiration as the cause of respiratory symptoms and complications. Thereby the possible effect of operation on the patient's respiratory symptoms is difficult to predict preoperatively.

Patients with regurgitation as the dominating symptom are often not helped with optimal medical treatment because regurgitation will persist even though there might be no acid production in the stomach. These patients have good results of anti-reflux surgery.

The occurrences of Barret's esophagus strengthen the indication for operation but are not an absolute indication for surgery by itself.

Surgical treatment may be considered when severe chronic reflux and:

- **No or incomplete effect of medical treatment**

- **Regurgitation as the primary symptom**

- **Complications to reflux disease (peptic strictures, Barrett)**

- **Lung problems probably caused by microaspirations**

- **The patient chooses not to get life-long medical treatment**

ENDOSCOPIC TREATMENT OF REFLUX DISEASE

The development within minimal invasive surgery has caused revision of normal treatment principles within a number of different diseases including the possibility of treating reflux by endoscopic procedures rather than laparoscopic procedures, meaning treatment with a gastroscope rather than with a laparoscope. There are currently 4 FDA (Food and Drug Administration) approved endoscopic procedures for the treatment of reflux disease:

- Endoscopic suturing (Bard Endocinch)
- EsophyX2 TIF Procedure (Transoral Incisionless Fundoplication Procedure)
- The NDO Surgical Endoscopic Plication System
- Local radio frequency treatment (Stretta)

At the endoscopic suturing technique 2-3 sutures are placed in the gastroesophageal transition zone and thereby local ischemia and secondary fibrosis are obtained in the area with a following reduction in the distal esophageal relaxations, increased distal esophageal pressure and thereby decreased reflux of acid from the stomach to the distal esophagus.

With the Stretta-method radiofrequency energy is applied from about 2 cm above the gastroesophageal transition zone to about 1.5 cm below. By this method there will be a reduction in the postprandial relaxation in the sphincter whereby reflux to the distal esophagus is decreased or hindered. Another mechanism could be local neurolysis whereby esophagus will be less sensitive to the acid thus causing fewer symptoms for the patient.

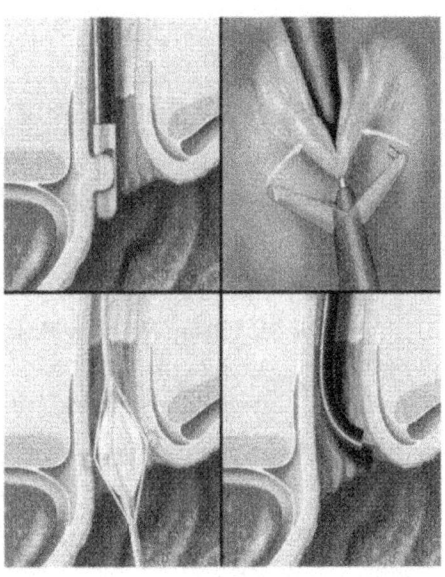

At the gastroplication procedure a full thickness suture is placed about 1 cm below the gastroesophageal transition zone. The method probably works by increasing the valve mechanism in the gastroesophageal transition zone at the same time as it probably reduces the compliance in the cardia/fundus region.

The preliminary results of all the techniques have shown that significant changes are obtained in the occurrence of heart burn, regurgitation and quality of life after endoscopic treatment. Many patients do not use proton pump inhibitors as long as 12 months after the treatment, but there does not seem to be convincing effects on the pH-values in the lower part of the esophagus. The exact mechanisms of action by the different endoscopic methods are more or less not known in detail and the final group of patients who will benefit from these new endoscopic treatments has therefore not yet been fully established.

The surgical (laparoscopic) treatment is, even though being minimal invasive, not without problems and the introduction of the endoscopic treatment alternatives will probably change the indications for treatment in the future.

Patients that have good symptom control, but do not want life-long proton pump inhibitor treatment may be a group suitable for endoscopic treatment.

Patients with changes in the motility in the esophagus (where it is not the tradition to recommend laparoscopic fundoplication) may be offered endoscopic treatment instead. The patients who previously have received laparoscopic operation but where there seem to be a recurrence of the reflux disease, may also be offered endoscopic treatment since the laparoscopic re-operation carries significant morbidity and even mortality.

Future physiological and clinical randomized trials will determine the final place in the treatment armamentarium for these new endoscopic procedures for patients with reflux disease. The data needed include of course effects on reflux symptoms as well as effects on long-term complications to reflux disease, quality of life, as well as health economic data.

PATIENT CASES FROM DAILY CLINICAL PRACTICE

36-year old woman with long anamnesis with "acid reflux", heartburn and retrosternal pain. No other diseases. Good effect of continuous proton pump inhibitor treatment in high dose, but the patient does not want life-long medical treatment.

Plan: Admit for surgical evaluation regarding the indication for laparoscopic anti-reflux surgery.

Examinations: Gastroscopy, esophagus manometry and 24-hours pH. After this a clinical consultation with a surgeon experienced in anti-reflux surgery.

30-year old man with a long anamnesis with periodical heartburn and "acid reflux". Long periods without symptoms and without the need for medication. In periods with symptoms he has good effect of proton pump inhibitor treatment.

Plan: The patient is informed of the reflux disease and the possibility of changes in life-style. Is informed about schedules for self-medication with proton pump inhibitors in periods with symptoms with short treatment regimens of a few days' duration and to stop when the symptoms have disappeared. Can also be informed about the use of antacids if symptoms are only light.

Investigations: None.

76-year old man with chronic alcohol use and many years of light reflux symptoms, but now also dysphagia and weight loss.

Plan: Malignant cause of the new symptom (dysphagia and weight loss) should be investigated very soon. Investigations: A gastroscopy showed a stricture 35 cm from the teeth. Biopsies were benign with normal epithelium.

Strategy: Balloon dilatation, maybe "repeated", and long-term treatment with proton-pump inhibitor, also if symptoms are not present.

55-year old woman with typical reflux disease for years, for long periods well-treated with moderate doses of proton pump inhibitors, but now also dysphagia.

Plan: Fast examination to find the cause of the newly

developed dysphagia.

Examinations: Gastroscopy showed a peptic stricture with benign biopsies.

Strategy: Balloon dilatation, maybe "repeated" and evaluation for possible laparoscopic fundoplication if the patient wants this. If she does not want surgery then continuous, probably life-long proton pump inhibitor treatment should be initiated.

35-year old singer, with increasing voice problems. Only slight upper dyspepsia, but a clinical suspicion of reflux disease.

Examinations: evaluation by an ENT (Ear, Nose, Throat) specialist. Gastroscopy, esophageus manometry and 24-hours pH.

Strategy: If pathological reflux is verified, then she should be referred to a surgeon for clinical consultation regarding the possibility for reflux surgery. The patient should be thoroughly informed about the possible effects of surgery on her voice problems since we cannot be sure, that surgery will actually help her even though she has pathological reflux.

55-year old women, with a 10 year history of various symptoms but primarily centered around dysphagia. Initially she had weight loss but she has had a stable weight for years now. Has undergone gastroscopy several times without pathological findings. She now comes with unclear symptoms with a weight loss of 12 kg, the production of big amounts of foam when coughing/throwing up every morning, and quite severe heartburn with no effect of proton pump inhibitors.

Examnations: Gastroscopy and esophagus manometry under the suspicion of achalasia.

Strategy: If achalasia is verified the patient will be offered laparoscopic operation with myotomy and fundoplication. Alternatively she may be offered one of the new endoscopic treatment alternatives.

ABOUT THE AUTHOR

Jacob Rosenberg (1964) was born and grew up in Copenhagen, Denmark. He is professor of surgery at the University of Copenhagen, and chief surgeon at the Gastro-unit, surgical section, Herlev Hospital (also in Copenhagen).

The author page at amazon.com is:
https://www.amazon.com/author/jacobrosenberg